COMPLETE GUIDE TO CARDIAC CHARACTERIZATION

A Comprehensive Manual To Advanced Techniques, Insights, Diagnostics, And Cutting-Edge Research In Cardiovascular Health

DR. BRUNO HORAN

Copyright © 2023 by Dr. Bruno Horan

All rights reserved. Except for brief quotations embodied in critical reviews and certain other noncommercial uses permitted by copyright law, no part of this publication may be reproduced, distributed, or transmitted in any form or by any means, Including photocopying, recording, or other electronic or mechanical methods, without the prior written permission of the publisher.

Disclaimer:

The information provided in this book, is intended for general informational purposes only and should not be considered as professional advice.

The author has made every effort to ensure the accuracy of the information presented. However, readers are advised to consult with a qualified healthcare professional before attempting any herbal remedies or making significant changes to their wellness routine. Individual health conditions vary, and what may be suitable for one person may not be appropriate for another.

It is important to note that the author is not in any endorsement deal, partnership, or affiliation with any organization, brand, or company mentioned in this book. Any references to specific products or services are based on the author's personal experience or general knowledge and do not imply an endorsement or promotion of those products or services

Contents

CONCERNING THIS BOOK

More than merely a medical work, "Cardiac Characterization: Unlocking the Secrets of Heart Health" serves as a compass to help both seasoned professionals and inquisitive minds navigate the complex pathways of the cardiovascular system. Fundamentally, this book is a lighthouse of information, explaining the basic features of the architecture and function of the heart and emphasizing how vital it is to preserve cardiac health.

Through a thorough analysis of cardiac disorders ranging from the ordinary to the complicated, readers are taken on a journey of discovery regarding the resilience and weaknesses of the heart. Understanding the significance of cardiac characterization in diagnosis enables people to see how specific instruments and methods become vital allies in solving cardiac riddles.

Step into the world of diagnostic tools, where the book walks you through the ins and outs of electrocardiograms, echocardiograms, and other devices that communicate with the heart. However, the importance of knowing the subtleties of the instruments, distinguishing between invasive and non-invasive techniques, and guaranteeing the highest level of safety throughout cardiac testing procedures cannot be overstated. After all, deft data interpretation becomes the pivot around which well-informed choices and efficient patient interaction are made.

About patients, the book skillfully negotiates the complexities of getting people ready for cardiac testing. In addition to gently addressing worries and minimizing dangers, it also highlights the significance of informed consent and cultivates a supportive atmosphere that promotes healing and understanding.

As the results begin to pour in, the book proves to be a reliable resource for understanding cardiac report language, differentiating between normal and abnormal findings, and compassionately conveying these facts. Every page reflects the values of inclusivity and individualized care, from addressing socioeconomic inequities to addressing pregnancy-related complexities and from addressing pediatric to geriatric issues.

Step inside the world of advanced imaging techniques. This book provides an introduction to cutting-edge technology and the moral ramifications associated with it. It's not only about looking to the present; wearable technology and artificial intelligence have the potential to completely transform cardiac diagnosis in the future.

Within the context of clinical practice, this book becomes more than just a compilation; it becomes a guide for facilitating the smooth integration of cardiac testing into patient care pathways, encouraging professional teamwork, and overcoming the challenges associated with standardization.

When the trip comes to an end, the book kindly answers often-asked questions and worries, easing fears, dispelling myths, and offering a lifeline of knowledge and assistance.

"Cardiac Characterization" is, in short, more than just a book; it's a monument to the art and science of cardiology, a celebration of the lifeblood of medicine, and a lighthouse that points patients and medical professionals in the direction of cardiac health.

An Overview of the Heart's Operations

As the body's pump, the heart is an essential component of the circulatory system that works nonstop to move blood throughout the body. It is separated into two ventricles and two atria, or four chambers. While the ventricles pump blood out of the heart, the atria receive blood. The heart prevents backflow by ensuring that blood flows in the proper direction through a sophisticated system of valves.

The heart's main job is to pump blood full of oxygen to the body's cells and organs while also expelling carbon dioxide and other waste. Maintaining the body's general health and functionality depends on this mechanism. The heart is also essential for controlling blood pressure and preserving the body's fluid balance.

The Value of Heart Health

Sustaining ideal heart health is essential for general health and lifespan. The many activities of the body are supported by effective blood circulation, which is ensured by a healthy heart. Severe problems, such as heart disease, heart attacks, and strokes, can result from poor cardiac health.

Heart health is influenced by several factors, including genetics, lifestyle choices, exercise, and diet. Heart health can be supported by eating a balanced diet high in fruits, vegetables, lean meats, and healthy grains. Frequent exercise enhances circulation, fortifies the heart muscle, and aids in blood pressure and weight management.

An Introduction to Heart Anatomy

To understand the heart's functioning and different cardiac diseases, one must have a basic understanding of its anatomy. The heart has four chambers: two atria and two ventricles, as was previously mentioned. To control blood flow, valves that open and close between these chambers are in place.

In addition, the pericardium, a sac that surrounds the heart, acts as a barrier against injury and friction caused by the heart's pumping motion. The coronary arteries, which supply the heart with its blood vessels, also guarantee that the heart muscle gets enough oxygen and nourishment.

Typical Heart Conditions

The structure and function of the heart can be impacted by a variety of cardiac disorders, from relatively modest problems to potentially fatal conditions. Among the prevalent heart ailments are:

Coronary artery disease (CAD): A disorder where plaque accumulates in the coronary arteries, reducing the amount of blood that reaches the heart muscle.

Heart failure is a disorder that causes weariness, breathlessness, and fluid retention because the heart cannot pump enough blood to meet the body's needs.

Arrhythmias: irregular heartbeats that can lead to chest discomfort, fainting, dizziness, and palpitations.

Damage or abnormalities to the heart's valves that impair blood flow and circulation are known as valvular heart disease.

A class of illnesses known as cardiomyopathies causes the heart muscle to grow, thicken, or stiffen.

Cardiac Characterization's Function in Diagnosis

When it comes to the diagnosis and treatment of different heart disorders, cardiac characterization is essential. It entails a thorough evaluation of the anatomy, physiology, and general health of the heart through the use of numerous diagnostic procedures and imaging modalities.

Typical techniques for characterizing the heart include:

An electrocardiogram, also known as an EKG or ECG, is a non-invasive diagnostic that captures the electrical activity of the heart to assist diagnose problems such as irregular heartbeats.

An echocardiogram is a type of ultrasonography that shows the chambers, valves, and blood flow of the heart in great detail.

Magnetic resonance imaging, or cardiac MRI, is an imaging method that creates incredibly detailed pictures of the anatomy and physiology of the heart, enabling accurate detection of cardiac disorders.

A minimally invasive treatment called cardiac catheterization entails putting a catheter into the heart to take blood samples, assess pressure, and do imaging tests.

Healthcare professionals can create a personalized treatment plan for each patient by precisely assessing the state of the heart. This could involve dietary adjustments, prescription drugs, surgery, or other treatments meant to strengthen the heart and avoid problems.

CHAPTER ONE

METHODS AND RESOURCES FOR CARDIAC DETAILING

Overview Of Diagnostic Instruments For Heart Characterization

Tools for diagnosis are essential for comprehending and evaluating cardiac health. The echocardiography and electrocardiogram (ECG) are two of the most often utilized instruments. These instruments offer important insights into the anatomy and physiology of the heart, assisting in the identification and management of a range of cardiac disorders.

ECG, or electrocardiogram

The non-invasive diagnostic technique known as an electrocardiogram, or ECG or EKG, is used to measure the electrical activity of the heart. Electrodes are applied to the skin to detect the electrical impulses produced by the heart's contractions and relaxations.

After that, these impulses are either digitally displayed or recorded on graph paper, enabling medical specialists to examine the heart's rhythm and spot any anomalies.

The conduction system, rhythm, and rate of the heart are all well-documented by the ECG. It is capable of identifying anomalies such as conduction problems, arrhythmias, and ischemia (inadequate blood supply to the heart muscle) symptoms. This information is essential for making the right treatment decisions and detecting a variety of heart problems.

Echocardiography

Echocardiography is a non-invasive imaging method that builds a precise image of the anatomy and function of the heart using sound waves. A transducer is applied to the chest during the process to produce images by emitting high-frequency sound waves (ultrasound) that reverberate off the heart. Healthcare professionals may see the heart's chambers, valves, and blood flow in real-time thanks to these photos.

Important details regarding the dimensions, morphology, and function of the heart can be learned using echocardiography. It is capable of identifying anomalies such as congenital cardiac defects, valve problems, and irregularities in heart activity. It can also identify heart failure symptoms and evaluate the heart's total pumping capacity (ejection fraction).

Methods That Are Invasive vs. Not

The difference between invasive and non-invasive cardiac characterization techniques is one of the most important ones. Non-invasive techniques, including electrocardiography and echocardiography, don't need to break through the skin or access any bodily cavities. Instead, they rely on outside sensors or imaging methods to obtain cardiac data.

Conversely, invasive techniques entail the insertion of tools or catheters into the body to gain direct access to the heart or blood vessels.

For more involved diagnostic procedures or interventions, including cardiac catheterization or electrophysiology tests, these techniques are frequently employed.

Invasive techniques can yield more thorough information, but they also come with a higher risk of consequences and call for specific tools and knowledge.

Safety Factors To Consider While Doing Cardiac Testing

To protect the patient's health during cardiac testing, safety must always come first. ECG and echocardiogram are examples of non-invasive testing. It is crucial to appropriately prepare the patient and adhere to standard guidelines for imaging and electrode placement. This lessens the patient's discomfort and risk while ensuring accurate findings.

Infection control, sterile technique, and monitoring for consequences like bleeding or arrhythmias are critical considerations for invasive operations. Healthcare professionals should be prepared to handle any unfavorable outcomes that may arise during the surgery and trained in emergency measures.

The Value Of Precise Data Interpretation

Making well-informed judgments regarding patient care requires accurate data interpretation. Healthcare professionals need to be able to distinguish between typical changes and abnormalities that could point to underlying heart pathology, whether they are interpreting echocardiography pictures or evaluating an ECG trace.

Inaccurate interpretation may result in an incorrect diagnosis or ineffective therapy, which could endanger the patient. To stay up to date with the latest developments in cardiac diagnostics and interpretation methods, healthcare professionals need to complete extensive training and ongoing education.

Healthcare professionals may give patients with heart diseases the best care possible, improving their quality of life and achieving better results, by using diagnostic tools wisely and correctly interpreting data.

CHAPTER TWO

GETTING READY FOR THE CARDIAC TEST

Guidelines For Patient Preparation

Patients must follow specific instructions before cardiac testing to guarantee accurate results and a seamless testing procedure.

First and foremost, patients need to adhere to any special directions given by their medical professionals concerning drug administration or dietary restrictions. This can entail going without food for a predetermined amount of time before the test or momentarily stopping any drugs that might affect the outcome.

Patients should also dress comfortably and refrain from wearing any accessories or jewelry that might need to be taken off during the testing process. Patients should also let their doctor know about any allergies or other medical conditions they may have, as this information can affect testing procedures and enable the medical staff to take the appropriate safety measures.

In addition, before the test, people should be ready to talk with their healthcare provider about any symptoms they may be having as well as their medical history. With the aid of this information, the testing procedure can be facilitated and the proper tests can be carried out to precisely evaluate the patient's cardiac condition.

Patients may help guarantee that their cardiac testing experience is as successful and efficient as possible by adhering to these preparation requirements, which will eventually result in better outcomes and more accurate diagnoses.

Possible Dangers And Issues

Patients should be informed of the risks and potential problems associated with cardiac testing techniques before undergoing any medical procedure. Even though the majority of cardiac tests are thought to be safe, patients should be aware of the hazards involved.

An allergic reaction to any drugs or contrast chemicals used during the procedure is one possible risk of cardiac testing. To prevent any negative responses, patients with known allergies should notify their healthcare provider before the test.

Another risk is experiencing pain or discomfort during the test, especially if it entails the insertion of catheters or other tools into the body. Nonetheless, medical professionals will take steps to reduce pain and guarantee the patient's comfort during the examination.

Certain cardiac tests may occasionally be associated with uncommon but potentially dangerous side effects, such as blood vessel damage or irregular heart rhythms. These issues are incredibly uncommon, though, and medical professionals will keep a careful eye on patients while they undergo testing to reduce the danger.

Overall, although cardiac testing carries certain possible dangers, the advantages of correctly identifying and treating heart diseases usually exceed the risks.

Before undergoing testing, patients should talk to their healthcare provider about any worries or inquiries they may have regarding the dangers associated with cardiac testing to make sure they are well-informed and at ease with the procedure.

Resolving Patient Issues

It is normal for people to feel anxious or worried before having cardiac testing, particularly if they have never had the procedure done before.

However, by offering clear guidance and assistance during the testing procedure, healthcare providers can help allay these worries and reduce anxiety.

Giving patients thorough explanations of the testing processes and what to anticipate at each stage of the process is one way to allay their fears. This can provide patients with a greater sense of control over their healthcare journey and demystify the testing process.

Healthcare professionals should also spend time listening to patients' worries and responding to any inquiries they may have. In the end, this can result in a more favorable testing experience by fostering a relationship of trust and rapport between patients and their healthcare providers.

It could also be advantageous for patients to bring a support person, like a friend or family member, to the testing appointment.

Having a familiar person by their side might offer comfort and emotional support during potentially difficult moments.

Healthcare professionals may guarantee that patients feel secure and at ease during cardiac testing by attending to their worries and offering assistance during the procedure. This will improve patient satisfaction and performance.

The Value Of Knowledgeable Consent

A crucial step in the cardiac testing process is informed consent, which guarantees that patients are aware of the advantages, disadvantages, and available options regarding the suggested testing procedures before they are carried out.

Before performing any medical procedures, including cardiac tests, healthcare professionals are required by law and ethics to get patients' informed consent.

Patients must be given thorough and unambiguous information about the intended testing methods, including the goal of the test, any possible risks or problems, and any alternate treatment choices that could be available, for their permission to be deemed informed.

Additionally, patients ought to be given the chance to clarify any areas of the testing procedure that they are unclear about and ask questions.

This gives patients the freedom to express any worries or desires they may have and enables them to make fully informed decisions regarding their healthcare.

Getting informed consent is an essential part of patient-centered care and also a legal requirement. Healthcare professionals can facilitate patients' sense of empowerment and engagement in their healthcare journeys by allowing them to participate in the decision-making process and honoring their autonomy.

Making Sure The Testing Environment Is Comfortable

Ensuring that patients receiving cardiac testing have a favorable experience requires creating a warm and inviting environment.

Healthcare professionals should make every effort to create a peaceful and encouraging testing atmosphere by paying attention to details like temperature, lighting, and noise levels.

Comfortable sitting and access to facilities like water and restrooms should be made available to patients. To further help patients feel less anxious and frustrated, healthcare practitioners should make sure that patients are seen promptly and that wait periods are kept to a minimum.

In addition, during the testing process, medical professionals should have open lines of communication with patients, going over each stage in detail and answering any queries or worries that may come up.

Patients may feel more comfortable and assured about the care they are getting as a result of this.

Healthcare professionals may guarantee that patients have a great experience during cardiac testing by putting their comfort and well-being first. This will ultimately improve results and raise patient satisfaction.

CHAPTER THREE

INTERPRETING THE RESULTS OF CARDIAC TESTS

Typical Versus Atypical Results

Making the distinction between normal and abnormal findings is essential when interpreting the results of cardiac tests. When tests are normal, the heart is usually healthy and not showing any symptoms of illness or discomfort.

These could include appropriate blood flow, regular rhythm, and a typical heart size. Conversely, abnormal results may indicate a variety of problems, ranging from minor ailments like arrhythmias to more significant difficulties like coronary artery disease or heart failure. Effective diagnosis and treatment of heart problems begin with the identification of these abnormalities.

A steady pulse on an electrocardiogram (ECG) or the absence of blockages in a coronary angiography are examples of normal findings that are frequently simple to understand. Unusual observations can include erratic heartbeats, high blood pressure inside the heart chambers, or anatomical anomalies including thickening of the wall or defective valves. To ascertain the relevance of any abnormal finding, it is necessary to consider the patient's symptoms and medical history.

Termology Often Used In Reports

Accurate interpretation requires knowledge of the terminology used in cardiac test reports. Words like "arrhythmia" describe any abnormal heartbeat, but "sinus rhythm" denotes a steady heartbeat originating from the sinus node. The term "ejection fraction" refers to the proportion of blood that the heart pumps out with each beat; normal ranges are between 55%

and 70%. A value in this range below can indicate cardiac failure.

Other widely used terminology are "hypertrophy," which describes the thickening of the heart muscle walls, and "ischemia," which denotes decreased blood flow to the heart muscle. "Regurgitation" is the term for heart valves that fail to seal properly, allowing blood to flow backward. "Stenosis" is the narrowing of the heart valves. Understanding these phrases can aid in understanding a patient's overall cardiac health.

Comprehending Parameters And Measurements

Heart test results frequently include a multitude of data and factors that must be comprehended. Heart rate, blood pressure, and cholesterol levels are important variables. Measurements such as end-diastolic volume (EDV) and left ventricular ejection fraction (LVEF) are crucial in an echocardiogram. The left ventricle's ability to pump blood with each contraction is measured by LVEF, whereas the ventricle's final filling volume is indicated by EDV.

Stress test metrics can reveal exercise capacity, such as the MET (metabolic equivalents) level, and ischemia can be detected by changes in the ST segment of an ECG. Heart biomarkers, such as troponin levels, are frequently measured in blood tests. These biomarkers rise in the event of myocardial infarction or heart attack, which is indicative of damage to the heart muscle. Gaining an understanding of these characteristics enables a thorough evaluation of heart health and function.

Recognizing Possible Warning Signs

Early intervention and treatment depend on the ability to recognize any warning signs in cardiac test findings. Extremely high or low heart rates, severe irregularities in blood pressure, or a markedly diminished ejection fraction are significant red flags.

An ejection fraction, for example, of less than 40% is highly suggestive of heart failure. Arrhythmias also need to be treated right away because they can be fatal, especially ventricular fibrillation or tachycardia.

Significant alterations in an ECG's ST segments, which could indicate acute ischemia, and elevated levels of cardiac enzymes like troponin, which might indicate recent heart muscle damage, are two further warning signs. Concerns should also be raised by unexplained hypertrophy or abrupt alterations in the anatomy and function of the heart on imaging examinations. These results require immediate, typically aggressive, diagnostic and treatment interventions.

Effectively Communicating Results To Patients

It is essential to properly convey cardiac test results to patients to gain their participation and comprehension of their treatment plan. Commence by outlining the test's objectives and typical outcomes. The results and their consequences should be explained in plain, non-technical terms. For example, rather than simply stating, "Your echocardiogram shows left ventricular hypertrophy," clarify, "The test shows that the muscle of your heart is thicker than normal, which can happen with high blood pressure."

It is imperative to be forthright about any alarming discoveries while offering comfort and a well-defined course of action. Allow the patient to ask questions and voice their concerns, and then clearly and empathetically answer them. Giving patients written summaries and visual aids—such as heart diagrams—can also aid in their understanding of complicated concepts. By helping them understand their disease and the required lifestyle modifications or medication, you can encourage them to take an active role in their treatment.

CHAPTER FOUR

CARDIAC CHARACTERISTICS DUE TO POPULATION CHANGES

Considerations For Cardiac Testing In Children

Diagnostic methods for children's heart health must be customized to take into consideration their distinct physiological traits.

For proper findings, pediatric patients frequently need specialized tools and procedures. For example, high-frequency ultrasound transducers are required during echocardiography to generate clear and detailed images due to the smaller size of their hearts. Additionally, as children's heart rates and rhythms differ greatly from adults', age-specific normal ranges must be taken into account when interpreting test results.

Furthermore, it is impossible to ignore the psychological component of pediatric testing. It's important to create a child-friendly environment because medical procedures can cause worry and terror in children.

Toys, movies, and child-life specialists can all be used to reduce their discomfort. For more intrusive examinations or for kids who can't stay still, sedation can be necessary. For parents to give informed permission and offer their kids adequate assistance, they must comprehend the goal and methodology of the tests.

Challenges In Geriatric Cardiac Assessment

Because of age-related physiological changes and the prevalence of comorbidities, cardiac evaluation in the elderly poses special obstacles. Chronic kidney disease, diabetes, and hypertension are among the many ailments that older adults frequently experience, which might make it more difficult to interpret heart testing. Furthermore, while assessing test results, age-related modifications like left ventricular hypertrophy and increasing arterial stiffness must be taken into account.

Challenges may also arise from functional restrictions and cognitive deficits in older people. For instance, mobility problems could make it difficult for them to complete exercise stress testing.

In certain situations, alternative testing techniques such as pharmacologic stress tests might be required. Older persons also frequently have polypharmacy, which necessitates a comprehensive examination of all drugs that may impact heart function or interfere with contrast agents used in imaging investigations.

Considering probable hearing or cognitive limitations, it is imperative to ensure efficient communication when working with elderly patients.

Accurate patient histories and test instructions can be obtained with the use of straightforward language and understanding checks.

Heart Testing While Expectant

Pregnancy-related cardiac testing must be carefully considered to safeguard the developing fetus as well as the mother.

Pregnancy-related physiological changes, such as elevated cardiac output and blood volume, must be considered as they may impact test results.

To reduce any possible risk to the fetus, non-invasive diagnostics such as Doppler ultrasonography and echocardiogram are recommended.

When required, some imaging modalities—like magnetic resonance imaging (MRI)—are regarded as safe to use while pregnant. Ionizing radiation is used in computed tomography (CT) scans and X-rays, however, it is usually avoided unless it is necessary.

Shielding strategies and reducing exposure are crucial if such tests are needed.

Managing cardiac problems that develop during gestation or those that already exist provides special challenges throughout pregnancy. To guarantee comprehensive care, cooperation with cardiologists and obstetricians who specialize in maternal-fetal medicine is essential. A comprehensive approach is necessary for the monitoring and management of disorders such as preeclampsia and peripartum cardiomyopathy to maximize the results for both mother and child.

Taking Socioeconomic And Cultural Aspects Into Account

Patient treatment and the characterization of the heart are significantly influenced by cultural and socioeconomic factors. Effective communication and patient compliance requires an understanding of and tolerance for cultural differences in views toward health, illness, and medical interventions. Certain cultural groups may hold certain ideas regarding the origins of cardiac disease or the best ways to treat it, for instance, and this may have an impact on their willingness to follow medical advice or submit to specific testing.

Another factor influencing access to cardiac testing and treatment is socioeconomic status. Individuals from less affluent socioeconomic origins may encounter obstacles including inadequate health insurance, problems with transportation, or restricted access to medical care. A multifaceted strategy is needed to overcome these obstacles, one that includes patient education, community engagement, and the provision of support services like financial aid and transportation.

Healthcare professionals should also be aware of the possibility of language hurdles and the requirement for translation services to guarantee effective contact with patients who do not understand the facility's primary language. Understanding the cultural background and being sensitive to the beliefs and behaviors of patients are just as important components of providing care that is culturally competent as language translation.

Adapting Testing Procedures To Various Populations

Age, gender, ethnicity, and medical history variations must be acknowledged and accommodated when designing cardiac testing methods for varied groups. For example, distinct heart diseases may manifest in men and women, requiring different diagnostic criteria and risk evaluations based on gender. For instance, women are more prone than men to develop unusual symptoms of cardiac disease. If normal male-centric criteria are employed, this could result in an underdiagnosis or misinterpretation.

Tailored treatments are also necessary due to ethnic disparities in illness prevalence and responsiveness to treatment. For instance, patients of African American descent may react differently to specific drugs and have a greater prevalence of hypertension. Personalized medicine is necessary because genetic variables can affect how well some diagnostic tests and treatments work.

Ensuring that all patients receive accurate diagnoses and successful treatments is ensured by developing and implementing protocols that take these variances into account.

To improve cardiac health outcomes for all groups, healthcare providers must receive ongoing education and training on the value of diversity and tailored care.

CHAPTER FIVE

SCIENTIFIC CARDIAC IMAGING METHODS

A Synopsis Of Advanced Imaging Techniques

Magnetic Resonance Imaging, or MRI

Strong magnets and radio waves are used in magnetic resonance imaging (MRI), a non-invasive procedure that produces finely detailed images of the heart and blood vessels.

MRI may produce high-resolution pictures of cardiac structures, such as the myocardium, valves, and pericardium, and is especially helpful for observing soft tissues.

When evaluating congenital cardiac disorders, scarring, and myocardial perfusion, this method is essential.

Computed Tomography, or CT

With Computed Tomography (CT), cross-sectional pictures of the heart and its surrounding components are created using X-rays.

For the evaluation of coronary artery disease, detailed pictures of the coronary arteries, calcium scoring, and plaque detection, cardiac computed tomography scans are very useful.

The diagnosis and treatment of coronary artery disease can be aided by the visualization of blood flow in the coronary arteries provided by CT angiography.

Positron Emission Tomography, or PET

A nuclear medicine procedure called Positron Emission Tomography (PET) evaluates the heart's metabolic and functional activities by using radioactive tracers. PET is very useful in evaluating inflammatory cardiac disorders, identifying viable myocardium, and detecting areas of diminished blood flow.

Understanding the metabolic activity of cardiac tissues is important for the diagnosis of diseases such as amyloidosis and sarcoidosis.

Signs And Symptoms Of Advanced Imaging

In several clinical situations, advanced cardiac imaging is recommended to give comprehensive anatomical and functional data. For evaluating cardiomyopathies, congenital heart disorders, and myocardial viability, for instance, cardiac MRI is recommended.

CT is frequently utilized in situations requiring quick imaging, pre-procedural planning for procedures, and the evaluation of coronary artery disease.

PET is recommended for determining the survivability of the myocardium after an infarction, monitoring myocardial perfusion, and identifying inflammatory diseases such as myocarditis.

Advantages And Drawbacks Of Every Method

Advantages

MRI: Provides detailed images of the anatomy and function of the heart without the use of ionizing radiation, and offers excellent soft tissue contrast. It works very well for assessing congenital cardiac abnormalities, identifying fibrosis, and describing cardiac tissue.

CT: Quick, high-definition imaging that works wonders for identifying calcifications and displaying coronary arteries. It works great for quickly determining the presence of coronary artery disease and scheduling interventional treatments.

PET: Provides distinct insights into the heart's metabolism and function, which are essential for the diagnosis and treatment of disorders like inflammatory diseases and myocardial ischemia. Its sensitivity and specificity in identifying cardiac viability are very good.

Restrictions

MRI: It can be difficult to get the patient to cooperate throughout longer scan times. Patients with extreme claustrophobia or those with specific metallic implant kinds should not get it.

CT: Uses ionizing radiation, which should be avoided if exposed frequently. It is less useful in patients with arrhythmias or rapid heartbeats and might not give as much information on soft tissue characteristics as magnetic resonance imaging (MRI).

PET: Its usage is restricted in some communities because it involves exposure to radioactive tracers. Furthermore, compared to MRI and CT, PET imaging has a lesser spatial resolution, and because it is a specialized modality, its availability may be restricted.

Analysis of Results from Advanced Imaging

Results from advanced cardiac imaging must be interpreted with specific knowledge and expertise. The interpretation of MRI results involves evaluating the heart's shape, function, and tissue properties. Anomalies related to wall motion, regions of delayed enhancement signifying fibrosis or scarring, and tissue characterization for ailments such as myocarditis or cardiomyopathies could be significant discoveries.

The coronary arteries are the main focus of CT results, which evaluate for plaques, calcifications, and stenosis. The degree of coronary artery disease can be determined in part by the calcium score, and a CT scan can show blood flow and arterial patency in great detail.

The distribution and strength of the radioactive tracer absorption are taken into consideration when interpreting PET results. Reduced uptake regions point to ischemia or infarction, whereas enhanced uptake regions may point to infection or inflammation. By distinguishing between a viable and non-viable myocardium, PET imaging is also utilized to evaluate the viability of the heart.

Including High-Tech Imaging In Clinical Practice

It takes a multidisciplinary team comprising nuclear medicine experts, radiologists, and cardiologists to incorporate sophisticated cardiac imaging into clinical practice. Procedures for selecting the best imaging modality for a given clinical situation should be developed.

For instance, if a patient has suspected coronary artery disease, a CT angiography may be performed to evaluate the coronary arteries first. If myocardial viability needs to be evaluated, a PET scan may then be performed.

When a patient has cardiomyopathy or suspected myocarditis, a cardiac MRI can be performed to assess function and offer a comprehensive tissue characterization.

To inform patient care, the results of advanced imaging examinations should be incorporated with clinical conclusions, test results from labs, and other diagnostic procedures. Frequent interdisciplinary conferences can help to ensure that imaging results are adequately incorporated into the treatment plan and can facilitate the discussion of complex cases.

CHAPTER SIX

NEW TECHNOLOGIES IN CHARACTERIZATION OF THE CARDIAC

Overview Of State-Of-The-Art Technologies

The field of cardiac characterization is undergoing rapid change because of technological breakthroughs that improve the accuracy and efficacy of heart disease diagnosis and treatment.

Advanced imaging methods that give precise images of the anatomy and function of the heart, such as cardiac MRI and 3D echocardiography, are among these state-of-the-art technologies.

Furthermore, the development of molecular imaging has made it possible to see the cellular and molecular functions occurring within the heart, providing previously unachievable insights.

In addition to increasing diagnostic precision, these technologies allow for individualized treatment regimens that are catered to the particular requirements of the patient.

The creation of high-resolution cardiac CT scans, which provide quicker and more comprehensive images while lowering the need for invasive treatments, is another noteworthy advancement.

These scans enable prompt interventions by rapidly identifying obstructions and other anomalies. Furthermore, by guaranteeing that patient data is freely accessible to healthcare practitioners, the integration of digital health records and telemedicine platforms promotes coordinated treatment and better outcomes.

Artificial Intelligence's Place In Heart Diagnostics

Artificial intelligence (AI) is revolutionizing cardiac diagnostics by offering strong instruments for the interpretation and analysis of data.

Large volumes of data from imaging tests, electronic health records, and wearable technology can be analyzed by AI algorithms, which can then spot trends and abnormalities that could be signs of cardiac disease.

For instance, machine learning models can use past data to forecast the chance of cardiac events in the future, allowing for proactive treatment and preventative measures.

AI improves the precision and efficacy of echocardiograms, MRIs, and CT scans in the field of imaging.

Automated devices can test cardiac function, detect structural anomalies promptly, and determine the severity of problems like cardiomyopathy or valve disease. This lowers the possibility of human error while simultaneously expediting the diagnosis procedure.

Additionally, AI-driven technologies that analyze electrocardiograms (ECGs) in real time and recommend the best course of treatment are being developed to help manage complex cardiac arrhythmias.

Wearable Technology For Ongoing Surveillance

With wearable technology providing a practical and non-invasive means of tracking heart function in real-time, wearables have become essential tools in the ongoing monitoring of cardiac health.

Heart rate, rhythm, and other critical factors can be measured by sensors built into devices like fitness trackers and smartwatches.

These wearables can identify anomalies like atrial fibrillation, alerting users to the need for medical care and offering early warnings.

Beyond simple heart rate monitoring, advanced wearables can measure blood pressure, measure oxygen saturation, and perform ECG functions. To better help consumers understand how lifestyle factors affect their heart health, several devices also track stress and activity. Wearables allow for continuous monitoring and the collecting of longitudinal data, which may be examined to spot trends and possible problems before they get out of hand. By empowering patients to take charge of their health, this proactive approach to cardiac care enables prompt interventions by medical professionals.

Possible Developments In The Future Of Cardiac Characterization

Future developments in cardiac characterization are expected to be shaped by several fascinating trends. The growing application of genetics and customized therapy in cardiology is one such development. Thanks to developments in genetic testing, inherited heart problems can now be identified and therapies can be tailored to a patient's unique genetic profile. This strategy could result in more focused and effective treatments, lower risk of negative side effects, and better patient outcomes.

The creation of implanted devices and bio-integrated sensors that provide continuous, real-time heart function monitoring is another new trend. In comparison to external wearables, these devices can offer more precise and thorough data, improving the capacity to identify and treat cardiac issues. Virtual and augmented reality technology will also soon be incorporated into cardiac care, providing cutting-edge patient education and engagement tools as well as immersive training for medical staff.

Ethics In The Acceptance Of New Technologies

We must address the ethical issues surrounding the introduction of new technology in cardiac characterization. Given the sensitive nature of health information gathered by wearables, artificial intelligence, and enhanced imaging, patient privacy and data security are crucial.

Maintaining patient trust and regulatory compliance requires making sure that data is transferred and maintained safely with strong security measures in place to prevent breaches.

Technology's propensity to widen health inequities is another ethical worry. The availability of state-of-the-art cardiac diagnostics and therapies may be restricted due to geographical location, socioeconomic status, and healthcare infrastructure. To guarantee that all patients may take advantage of the most recent improvements in cardiac care, efforts must be made to guarantee equal access to these developments. To promote trust and understanding between patients and healthcare professionals, it is also essential that AI and machine learning be used transparently, with clear communication about how these tools are utilized in diagnosis and treatment.

CHAPTER SEVEN

CHARACTERIZATION OF THE CARDIAC IN CLINICAL PRACTICE

Including Cardiovascular Testing In Patient Care Routines

To guarantee prompt and reliable diagnosis of cardiovascular illnesses, cardiac testing must be smoothly integrated into patient care pathways. The first step in the procedure is to identify patients who are at risk by doing screenings and regular checkups.

For instance, first non-invasive procedures such as ECG, echocardiography, or stress testing should be given priority to patients presenting with chest pain or those with a history of hypertension and diabetes. Patients will find it more convenient and hospital congestion will be reduced if these tests are conducted in outpatient settings.

Furthermore, it's critical to establish precise protocols for determining when to proceed to more sophisticated imaging modalities like cardiac MRI or CT angiography.

These recommendations should be customized for each patient's unique profile, taking into account things like age, co-occurring conditions, and the outcomes of the first tests.

To rule out coronary artery disease, for example, a patient with an unsatisfactory stress test result could be referred for a CT angiography.

To further streamline the procedure and guarantee that no patient is overlooked, it is possible to integrate electronic health records (EHR) for tracking test results and follow-up consultations.

For cardiac characterization to be effective, healthcare practitioners must work together. To provide complete care, cardiologists, general practitioners, radiologists, and nurses collaborate.

Frequent meetings of multidisciplinary teams can help to promote the discussion of complex situations by providing a forum for expert viewpoints and a range of contributions.

For instance, to choose the most effective course of treatment and diagnosis, a patient with a suspected myocardial infarction may profit from the joint expertise of an interventional radiologist and a cardiologist.

To make sure that everyone in the team is up to date on the most recent developments in cardiac diagnostics, training, and ongoing education are provided. For example, primary care doctors can receive training to identify potential cardiac problems early and know when to send patients for specialized testing.

 Further improving patient outcomes is the implementation of a coordinated care approach, in which nurses oversee patient follow-ups and guarantee adherence to recommended diagnostic protocols.

Case Studies Showing How Beneficial Cardiac Characterization Is

Case studies are useful for showing how cardiac characterization can be applied in real-world scenarios. A 55-year-old man who has a history of smoking and hypertension and who presents with unusual chest pain could serve as an example of this situation.

The patient may have a normal initial ECG and blood tests, but stress echocardiography indicates anomalies in the region of wall motion, which prompts a coronary angiography that finds severe blockages.

A successful angioplasty is the result of prompt intervention via proper cardiac characterization, underscoring the potentially life-saving value of comprehensive diagnostic methods.

A teenage athlete who experiences unexplained fainting spells could be the subject of another case. It's possible that a basic medical examination and testing will turn up nothing wrong

. On the other hand, sophisticated cardiac MRI may detect an uncommon illness like arrhythmogenic right ventricular cardiomyopathy (ARVC).

This diagnosis demonstrates how sophisticated cardiac characterization methods can identify diseases that might otherwise go undetected until it's too late and enable appropriate care and preventive measures.

Implementing Standardized Protocols Presents Difficulties

There are various obstacles to overcome while implementing standardized techniques for cardiac characterization. The variation in resources available in various healthcare settings is one of the main challenges. For example, rural clinics may not even have access to basic diagnostic instruments, while urban hospitals may have cutting-edge imaging technology. This discrepancy may result in uneven patient care and inconsistent procedure application.

Healthcare professionals' aversion to change because they may be used to set routines is another difficulty. Strong training initiatives and data-and case study-based demonstrations of the advantages of standardized methods are necessary to overcome this. In addition, it might be challenging to maintain protocol adherence in a busy, fast-paced clinical setting. This problem can be lessened by creating user-friendly guidelines and adding decision-support capabilities to EHR systems.

Methods For Improving Heart Diagnostic Services

Several calculated strategies are needed to optimize cardiac diagnostic services. Creating specialized cardiac diagnostic centers within larger hospitals is one useful tactic. These facilities may provide specialist testing and knowledgeable result interpretation, guaranteeing top-notch medical care. For instance, a cardiac MRI center can offer more precise and thorough imaging, which improves diagnostic results.

Another crucial tactic is to fund healthcare providers' ongoing professional development. Staff members can stay knowledgeable and skilled by attending frequent workshops and seminars on the newest diagnostic methods and technology. Finding areas for improvement can also be aided by establishing a culture of continuous quality improvement through frequent audits and feedback loops.

Technology utilization is also essential for optimization. By using telemedicine to provide virtual consultations, cardiac doctors can reach underprivileged communities. Analyzing diagnostic data with artificial intelligence can also improve efficiency and accuracy, lessening the burden on human clinicians and expediting the diagnosis process. To ensure that patients obtain timely and correct diagnoses, AI systems, for example, can immediately discover trends in ECGs or imaging investigations that would be missed by the human eye.

CHAPTER EIGHT

RESOLVING COMMON QUESTIONS AND FAQS

Controlling Cardiac Test-Related Anxiety

Anxiety before cardiac testing is rather common. It's crucial to keep in mind that these examinations are intended to offer insightful data regarding your cardiac health, which may eventually result in more effective preventative and treatment measures.

Try using relaxation methods like deep breathing, meditation, or visualization to help you control your anxiety.

Speaking with your healthcare practitioner about your worries can also help allay anxiety and offer assurance regarding the testing procedure. Recall that your healthcare team is at your side at every turn, so never feel alone.

Talking About Money Issues And Insurance Coverage

Although navigating the financial implications of cardiac testing might be challenging, assistance is available. Examine your insurance policy first to find out which tests are covered and whether there are any additional fees or copayments. Do not hesitate to discuss any concerns you may have regarding affordability with a financial counselor at the hospital or clinic where you will be receiving testing, or with your healthcare physician. They can assist in looking into alternate testing procedures that can be more cost-effective, as well as payment choices and financial assistance programs.

Dispelling Myths Regarding Cardiac Testing

Heart testing is the subject of numerous myths and misconceptions, which may cause unwarranted fear or reluctance. The idea that all cardiac examinations are intrusive or uncomfortable is often held. Many tests are painless and non-invasive, like echocardiograms and electrocardiograms (ECGs). Another myth is that people with known heart issues or older persons are the only ones who require cardiac testing. All ages, however, may benefit from cardiac testing, particularly if risk factors, such as high blood pressure or a family history of heart disease, are present.

Managing Difficulties And Unfavorable Responses

Adverse responses or problems might happen during or after cardiac testing, however they are uncommon. It's critical to be informed about potential hazards and to share any worries you may have with your healthcare professional. It is important to report symptoms right once, including dizziness, shortness of breath, and chest pain. Most of the time, medical professionals are ready to handle any issues with promptness and efficiency. You can reduce the possibility of unfavorable outcomes and guarantee a secure testing procedure by taking proactive measures and being watchful of your health.

Supplying Resources For More Data And Assistance

You might need more assistance or have more questions after having cardiac tests. Thankfully, there are lots of tools at your disposal to support you on your road toward heart health. For trustworthy information and resources, think about getting in touch with groups like the American Heart Association or the National Heart, Lung, and Blood Institute. An additional resource for a feeling of community and connection with those going through similar situations is online forums and support groups. You should always keep in mind that information is power, so arming yourself with it can help you make decisions about your heart health both now and in the future.

www.ingramcontent.com/pod-product-compliance
Lightning Source LLC
Chambersburg PA
CBHW051914250726
48659CB00002B/639